High protein plant based diet cookbook for Beginners

Tasty, Quick, Delicious recipe for athletes, men, women and for weight loss.

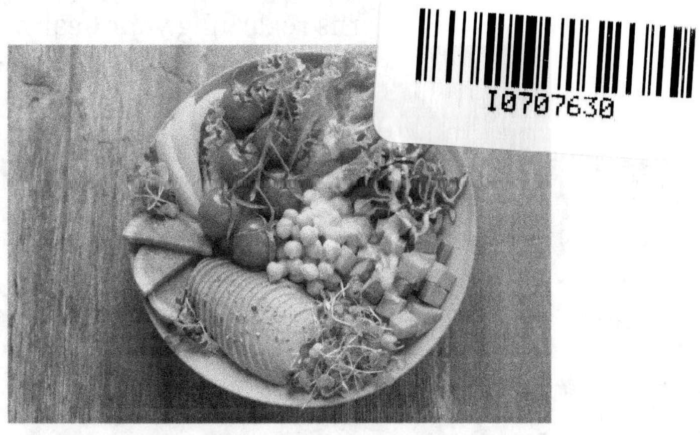

Paula A. Nicholas

The information in this book is provided for educational purposes only and is not intended as a substitute for professional medical advice, diagnosis, or treatment. Please seek the advice of a qualified health care professional if you have any questions or concerns regarding your health. The author and publisher specifically disclaim any liability, loss, or risk that may be incurred as a result of the use and application of the information contained in this book.

<u>Table of Content</u>

Overview of plant-based diets
Benefits of a vegan diet.

Essential Nutrients for Athletes on a Vegan Diet
Protein sources and requirements
Iron, calcium, and other key minerals
Omega-3 fatty acids and vitamin B12 supplementation

High-protein breakfast options
Plant-based protein smoothies

Energy-boosting breakfasts
Energy-boosting breakfasts tips
Snacks to fuel long training sessions
Recovery Meals for Vegan Athletes

Hydration Strategies for Vegan Athletes
Importance of hydration in athletic

Plant-powered celebratory meals
Desserts and treats for special occasions.

Conclusion

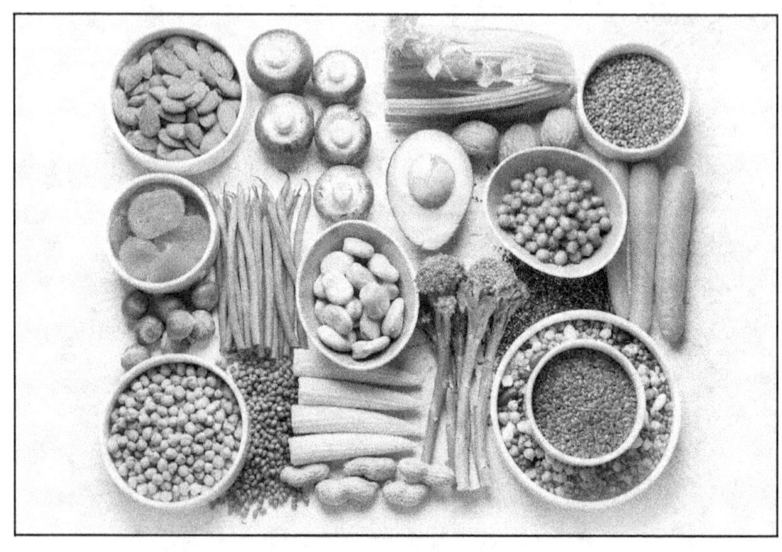

Chapter 1

Overview of plant based diet

A plant-based diet comprises foods such as fruits, vegetables, grains, legumes, nuts, seeds, and plant-based oils that are predominantly sourced from plants. While the nature and limits of plant-based diets can vary greatly, generally speaking, they decrease or completely eliminate the intake of animal products including meat, dairy, eggs, and fish.

 A plant-based diet brings the following:

Whole, minimally processed foods are the mainstay of plant-based diets. A large range of fruits, vegetables, whole grains, legumes, nuts, and seeds are included in this. These foods support general health and wellbeing since they are high in fiber, antioxidants, phytochemicals, and important minerals.

Variety and balance

The concepts of balance and diversity are essential to a plant-based diet. Incorporating a wide variety of plant-based foods guarantees a wide range of nutrients and tastes, while ensuring that macronutrients (proteins, fats, and carbs) are balanced to fulfill specific dietary demands.

Cutbacks or Removal of Animal Products:

Plant-based diets usually include cutting back on or eliminating the intake of meat, poultry, fish, dairy products, and eggs, while they do not always call for the total removal of animal products. Some people could decide to sometimes consume modest amounts of animal products, while others follow a strict vegan diet that forbids eating anything that comes from animals.

Advantages for Health:

Plant-based diets have been linked to a host of health advantages, including a lower risk of obesity, type 2 diabetes, heart disease, and several malignancies. Compared to omnivorous diets, they usually have higher levels of fiber, vitamins, minerals, and antioxidants and lower levels of cholesterol and saturated fat.

Sustainability of the Environment:

Plant-based diets are frequently advocated because they are sustainable for the environment.
Plant-based food production often uses less natural resources, emits fewer greenhouse gases, and has a less environmental impact than animal agriculture. Eating a plant-based diet can help protect natural resources and slow down the effects of climate change.

Questions for thought

1. What are your thoughts considering Vegan meal and what made you stick to this diet?

2. How has it also sharpened you?

____

____

____

____

____

____

____

____

Chapter 2

Essential Nutrients for Athletes on a Vegan Diet

Protein:

Plant-based protein sources include legumes (beans, lentils, chickpeas), tofu, tempeh, edamame, quinoa, nuts, seeds, and whole grains. Consuming a variety of these foods throughout the day ensures sufficient protein intake.

Vitamin B12:

Vitamin B12 is primarily found in animal products, so it's important for vegans to obtain it from fortified foods or supplements. Fortified plant-based milk, breakfast cereals, and nutritional yeast are common sources.

Iron:

Plant-based iron sources include lentils, beans, tofu, tempeh, dark leafy greens (spinach, kale), fortified cereals, and whole grains. Consuming vitamin C-rich foods alongside iron-rich foods can enhance iron absorption.

Calcium:

Good plant-based calcium sources include fortified plant milks (soy, almond, oat), tofu, tempeh, leafy greens (kale, collard greens, bok choy), and fortified orange juice. Calcium absorption can be influenced by the presence of oxalates and phytates in some plant foods.

Omega-3 Fatty Acids:

Sources of omega-3 fatty acids for vegans include flaxseeds, chia seeds, hemp seeds, walnuts, and algae-based supplements. These provide alpha-linolenic acid (ALA), which the body can convert into EPA and DHA, although conversion rates can be limited.

Vitamin D:

Vitamin D is mainly obtained through sunlight exposure. For those with limited sun exposure, vitamin D2 or vitamin D3 supplements derived from lichen (for D3) can be used. Fortified plant-based milks and cereals may also contain vitamin D.

Zinc:

Plant-based zinc sources include legumes, nuts, seeds, whole grains, and tofu. Phytates in plant foods can bind to zinc, so consuming a variety of zinc-rich foods is important. Soaking, fermenting, or sprouting can also enhance zinc absorption.

Iodine:

Iodine-rich foods include seaweed, iodized salt, and certain vegetables grown in iodine-rich soils. If these sources are insufficient, an iodine supplement or iodine-containing multivitamin may be considered.

Vitamin A:

Beta-carotene, found in orange and yellow vegetables (carrots, sweet potatoes, butternut squash) and dark leafy greens (kale, spinach), is a precursor to vitamin A. Vegans can obtain sufficient vitamin A from these plant sources.

Fiber:

A vegan diet rich in fruits, vegetables, whole grains, legumes, nuts, and seeds provides ample dietary fiber. Fiber is essential for digestive health and helps maintain stable blood sugar levels.

All of these are the necessary nutrients for a vegan diet.

Questions
Has this nutrients been incorporated in your diet?
How much do you take fruits high in protein such
as Guava, Avocado, Blackberries?

Chapter 3

High-protein breakfast options

Vegan Tofu Scramble:

Sauté crumbled tofu with veggies like bell peppers, onions, and spinach. Season with turmeric, black salt, and herbs.

Chickpea Flour Omelette:

Mix chickpea flour with water, turmeric, baking powder, and veggies to make a protein-packed omelette.

Quinoa Breakfast Bowl:

Cook quinoa and top it with sliced almonds, berries, chia seeds, and nut butter.

Vegan Protein Pancakes:

Combine whole wheat or oat flour with plant-based protein powder, almond milk, and vanilla extract to make pancakes.

Tempeh Bacon Avocado Toast:

Toast whole-grain bread and top it with sliced avocado and tempeh bacon.

Vegan Breakfast Burrito:

Fill a tortilla with black beans, sautéed veggies, avocado, and salsa.

Vegan Protein Muffins:

Make muffins using a combination of whole wheat flour, plant-based protein powder, and mashed bananas.

High-Protein Overnight Oats:

Mix rolled oats with plant-based protein powder, chia seeds, and almond milk. Refrigerate overnight and top with fruit in the morning.

Vegan Breakfast Burrito Bowl:

Combine quinoa, black beans, sautéed veggies, avocado, and salsa for a hearty breakfast bowl.

Chickpea and Spinach Breakfast Hash:

Sauté chickpeas with spinach, cherry tomatoes, and spices for a flavorful and protein-rich breakfast hash.

Vegan Protein Waffles:

Make waffles using a batter of plant-based protein powder, almond milk, and a touch of baking powder.

Vegan Tofu Benedict:

Top an English muffin with sautéed spinach, tomato slices, and a vegan hollandaise sauce made from silken tofu.

Protein-Packed Acai Bowl:

Blend acai berries with plant-based protein powder, frozen fruit, and almond milk. Top with granola and sliced almonds.

Vegan Chickpea and Vegetable Frittata:

Bake a frittata with chickpea flour, veggies, and spices for a protein-rich breakfast.

Almond Butter and Banana Sandwich:

Spread almond butter on whole-grain bread and add sliced banana for a simple yet satisfying breakfast.

Vegan Spinach and Mushroom Breakfast Wrap:

Sauté spinach and mushrooms, wrap them in a whole-grain tortilla with hummus, and enjoy a savory breakfast wrap.

Plant-based protein smoothies

Berry Protein Blast:

Ingredients:
1 cup mixed berries (strawberries, blueberries, raspberries)
1 banana
1 scoop plant-based protein powder
1 cup almond milk
Ice cubes

Method: Blend all ingredients until smooth.

Tropical Green Protein Smoothie:

Ingredients:
1 cup pineapple chunks
1/2 mango, diced
Handful of spinach
1 scoop plant-based protein powder
1 cup coconut water

Method: Blend until creamy and enjoy the tropical goodness.

Peanut Butter Banana Protein Smoothie:

Ingredients:
2 ripe bananas
2 tablespoons peanut butter
1 scoop plant-based protein powder
1 cup almond milk
Ice cubes

Method: Blend until smooth and creamy.

Chocolate Almond Protein Shake:

Ingredients:
1 cup almond milk

1 scoop chocolate plant-based protein powder
1 tablespoon almond butter
Ice cubes

Method: Blend until well combined for a rich and chocolaty shake.

Mint Chocolate Chip Protein Smoothie:

Ingredients:
1 cup spinach
1 scoop chocolate plant-based protein powder
1/2 teaspoon peppermint extract
1 tablespoon cacao nibs
1 cup almond milk

Method: Blend until smooth, and enjoy the refreshing minty flavor.

Coffee Protein Smoothie:

Ingredients:
1 cup brewed coffee, cooled
1 scoop plant-based protein powder
1 banana
1 tablespoon almond butter
Ice cubes

Method: Blend until creamy for a caffeinated protein boost.

Vanilla Berry Protein Smoothie:

Ingredients:
1 cup mixed berries (strawberries, blueberries, raspberries)
1 scoop vanilla plant-based protein powder
1 cup oat milk
Ice cubes

Method: Blend until smooth and enjoy the sweet and fruity combination.

Green Protein Power Smoothie:

Ingredients:
1 cup kale or spinach
1/2 cucumber, peeled
1/2 green apple
1 scoop plant-based protein powder
1 cup coconut water

Method: Blend until the greens are well incorporated for a nutrient-packed smoothie.

Cherry Almond Protein Shake:

Ingredients:
1 cup frozen cherries
1 scoop vanilla plant-based protein powder
1 tablespoon almond butter
1 cup almond milk

Method: Blend until smooth and enjoy the cherry-almond goodness.

Mango Turmeric Protein Smoothie:

Ingredients:
1 cup mango chunks
1 scoop plant-based protein powder
1/2 teaspoon turmeric powder
1 tablespoon chia seeds
1 cup coconut water

Method: Blend until creamy for a tropical and anti-inflammatory smoothie.

Protein-rich salads and bowls

Quinoa and Chickpea Salad Bowl:

Ingredients:

Cooked quinoa
Chickpeas (canned or cooked)
Cherry tomatoes, halved
Cucumber, diced
Red onion, finely chopped
Fresh parsley, chopped
Olive oil and lemon dressing
Salt and pepper to taste

Method:
In a bowl, combine cooked quinoa, chickpeas, tomatoes, cucumber, red onion, and parsley.
Drizzle with olive oil and lemon dressing, and season with salt and pepper.
Toss the ingredients well and enjoy a protein-packed quinoa and chickpea salad.

Lentil and Roasted Vegetable Salad:

Ingredients:
Cooked lentils (green or brown)
Roasted sweet potatoes
Roasted Brussels sprouts
Mixed greens
Avocado, sliced
Balsamic vinaigrette
Toasted pumpkin seeds

Method:
Mix cooked lentils with roasted sweet potatoes,
Brussels sprouts, and mixed greens.
Top with sliced avocado and drizzle with balsamic
vinaigrette.
Sprinkle toasted pumpkin seeds for added crunch
and protein.

Chickpea and Avocado Salad:

Ingredients:
Canned chickpeas, drained and rinsed
Cherry tomatoes, halved
Cucumber, diced
Red bell pepper, diced
Avocado, diced
Fresh cilantro, chopped
Lime juice
Olive oil
Salt and pepper to taste

Method:
In a bowl, combine chickpeas, tomatoes, cucumber,
bell pepper, avocado, and cilantro.
Drizzle with lime juice and olive oil, and season
with salt and pepper.
Gently toss the ingredients to create a refreshing
and protein-rich chickpea and avocado salad.

Tofu and Edamame Buddha Bowl:

Ingredients:
Baked or pan-fried tofu cubes
Edamame, steamed
Quinoa or brown rice
Shredded carrots
Purple cabbage, thinly sliced
Avocado, sliced
Sesame ginger dressing
Sesame seeds for garnish

Method:
Arrange cooked quinoa or brown rice in a bowl.
Add baked or pan-fried tofu, steamed edamame, shredded carrots, purple cabbage, and sliced avocado.
Drizzle with sesame ginger dressing and sprinkle sesame seeds on top.

Black Bean and Corn Salad Bowl:

Ingredients:
Canned black beans, drained and rinsed
Corn kernels (fresh or thawed if frozen)
Red onion, finely chopped
Cherry tomatoes, halved

Fresh cilantro, chopped
Lime juice
Olive oil
Cumin and chili powder
Salt and pepper to taste

Method:
Combine black beans, corn, red onion, tomatoes,
and cilantro in a bowl.
In a small bowl, whisk together lime juice, olive oil,
cumin, chili powder, salt, and pepper to create a
dressing.
Pour the dressing over the salad and toss gently.
Enjoy this flavorful and protein-rich black bean and
corn salad.

Chapter 4

Energy boosting diet for athletes

Breakfast: Protein-Packed Smoothie Bowl

Ingredients:

1 scoop plant-based protein powder
1 cup mixed berries (blueberries, strawberries, raspberries)
1 banana
1 tablespoon almond butter
1 tablespoon chia seeds
1 cup almond milk

Method:

Blend all ingredients until smooth.
Pour into a bowl and top with granola, sliced almonds, and a drizzle of agave syrup.

<u>Mid-Morning Snack: Oatmeal and Fruit</u>

Ingredients:

1 cup cooked oats
1 tablespoon hemp seeds

1 tablespoon maple syrup
Sliced bananas and berries for topping

Method:

Mix hemp seeds into the cooked oats.
Top with sliced bananas, berries, and a drizzle of maple syrup.

Lunch: Quinoa and Chickpea Salad Bowl

Ingredients:

1 cup cooked quinoa
1 cup chickpeas (canned, drained, and rinsed)
Mixed greens (spinach, kale)
Cherry tomatoes, cucumber, and red onion
Avocado slices
Lemon-tahini dressing

Method:

Combine quinoa, chickpeas, mixed greens, and chopped vegetables in a bowl.
Top with avocado slices and drizzle with lemon-tahini dressing.

Afternoon Snack: Trail Mix and Fresh Fruit

Ingredients:

Handful of raw nuts (almonds, walnuts, cashews)
Dried fruits (apricots, figs, dates)
Fresh apple slices

Method:

Mix nuts and dried fruits to create a trail mix.
Enjoy with fresh apple slices for a quick and
energizing snack.

Dinner: Sweet Potato and Black Bean Burrito Bowl

Ingredients:

Roasted sweet potatoes
Black beans (canned, drained, and rinsed)
Brown rice or quinoa
Sautéed bell peppers and onions
Fresh salsa
Guacamole

Method:

Assemble the bowl with brown rice or quinoa, black beans, roasted sweet potatoes, sautéed vegetables, fresh salsa, and guacamole.

Evening Snack: Protein-Packed Chia Pudding

Ingredients:

2 tablespoons chia seeds
1 cup almond milk
1 tablespoon almond butter
Berries for topping

Method:

Mix chia seeds with almond milk and let it sit in the refrigerator until it thickens.
Top with almond butter and fresh berries.

Hydration Throughout the Day:

Drink plenty of water throughout the day to stay hydrated.
Consider coconut water for added electrolytes, especially after intense workouts.

Additional Tips:

Ensure an adequate intake of iron, calcium, vitamin B12, omega-3 fatty acids, and vitamin D through fortified foods or supplements if needed.
Adjust portion sizes based on individual energy needs and activity levels.
Include a variety of colorful fruits and vegetables to get a broad spectrum of vitamins and minerals.

Snacks to fuel long training sessions

Chickpea and Avocado Toast:

Ingredients:
Whole-grain bread slices
Mashed avocado
Seasoned chickpeas (canned or roasted)
Optional: Sprinkle of nutritional yeast, chili flakes

Instructions:
Toast the whole-grain bread slices.
Spread mashed avocado on the toast.
Top with seasoned chickpeas.
Optionally, add a sprinkle of nutritional yeast or chili flakes for extra flavor.

Nutritional Benefits: This snack provides a combination of healthy fats from avocado, complex carbohydrates from whole-grain bread, and protein from chickpeas.

Trail Mix with Nuts and Dried Fruits:

Ingredients:
Mixed nuts (almonds, walnuts, cashews)
Dried fruits (apricots, figs, raisins)
Seeds (pumpkin seeds, sunflower seeds)
Dark chocolate chunks or cacao nibs

Instructions:
Mix equal parts of nuts, dried fruits, and seeds in a bowl.
Add dark chocolate chunks or cacao nibs for a sweet touch.
Portion into snack-sized containers for convenient, on-the-go munching.

Hummus and Veggie Sticks:

Ingredients:
Hummus (store-bought or homemade)
Carrot sticks, cucumber slices, bell pepper strips

Instructions:
Arrange a variety of veggie sticks on a plate.

Dip them in hummus for a satisfying and nutritious snack.

Nutritional Benefits: Hummus provides protein and healthy fats, while the veggies offer vitamins, minerals, and fiber.

Vegan Protein Smoothie:

Ingredients:
Plant-based protein powder
Almond milk or any plant-based milk
Banana
Frozen berries (strawberries, blueberries)
Optional: Nut butter or chia seeds

Instructions:
Blend all ingredients until smooth.
Pour into a shaker bottle or a portable cup for a quick, protein-packed drink.
Nutritional Benefits: This smoothie delivers a combination of protein, carbohydrates, and antioxidants.

Vegan Energy Bars:

Ingredients:
Rolled oats

Almond butter
Agave syrup or maple syrup
Plant-based protein powder
Dried fruits (dates, figs)

Instructions:
Blend rolled oats, almond butter, agave syrup, and plant-based protein powder in a food processor.
Add chopped dried fruits and pulse until well combined.
Press the mixture into a lined pan and refrigerate until firm.
Cut into bars or squares for a convenient, homemade energy snack.

Nutritional Benefits: These energy bars offer a balanced profile of carbohydrates, protein, and healthy fats for sustained energy.

Recovery Meals for Vegan Athletes

Chickpea and Sweet Potato Curry:

Ingredients:
Chickpeas (canned, drained, and rinsed)
Sweet potatoes, diced
Spinach or kale

Coconut milk
Curry spices (turmeric, cumin, coriander)

Instructions:
Cook chickpeas, sweet potatoes, and greens in a curry sauce made with coconut milk and spices.

Vegan Lentil and Vegetable Stew:

Ingredients:
Lentils (green or brown)
Carrots, celery, and onions
Vegetable broth
Garlic and herbs

Instructions:
Simmer lentils and vegetables in vegetable broth with garlic and herbs for a hearty stew.

Tofu and Vegetable Stir-Fry with Brown Rice:

Ingredients:
Tofu, cubed
Mixed vegetables (broccoli, bell peppers, snap peas)
Tamari or soy sauce
Brown rice

Instructions:
Stir-fry tofu and vegetables in tamari or soy sauce and serve over brown rice.

Pasta with Lentil Bolognese:

Ingredients:
Whole-grain or lentil pasta
Lentils (cooked or canned)
Tomato sauce
Garlic, onions, and Italian herbs

Instructions:
Sauté garlic and onions, add cooked lentils and tomato sauce, and serve over pasta.

Vegan Buddha Bowl:

Ingredients:
Quinoa or brown rice
Roasted sweet potatoes
Steamed kale or spinach
Avocado slices
Tahini dressing

Instructions:

Assemble a bowl with quinoa, roasted sweet potatoes, steamed greens, and top with avocado and tahini dressing.

Vegan Chili with Beans and Vegetables:

Ingredients:
Mixed beans (kidney, black, pinto)
Diced tomatoes
Bell peppers, onions, and garlic
Chili spices (cumin, chili powder, paprika)

Instructions:
Simmer mixed beans, tomatoes, and vegetables with chili spices for a hearty vegan chili.

Vegan Protein Smoothie:

Ingredients:
Plant-based protein powder
Banana
Frozen berries
Almond milk

Instructions:
Blend plant-based protein powder, banana, berries, and almond milk for a quick and easy recovery smoothie.

Questions
Write down other delicious vegan smoothies you love

____

____

____

____

____

____

____

Don't forget to make them..

<u>Chapter 5</u>

<u>*Hydration Strategies for Vegan Athletes*</u>

Hydration is crucial for all athletes, including those following a vegan diet. Here are some hydration strategies specifically tailored for vegan athletes:

Water Intake:

Ensure you are drinking enough water throughout the day. The general recommendation is to aim for at least 8 cups (64 ounces) of water daily, but individual needs can vary based on factors such as activity level, climate, and body weight.

Electrolyte Balance:

Vegan athletes, like any other athletes, need to maintain electrolyte balance. While electrolytes are often associated with sports drinks, there are vegan-friendly options available. Coconut water is a natural source of electrolytes, providing potassium and sodium. You can also consider plant-based electrolyte supplements.

Incorporate Hydrating Foods:

Consume hydrating foods that have high water content. Fruits and vegetables such as watermelon, cucumber, oranges, strawberries, and celery are excellent choices. These foods not only contribute to your fluid intake but also provide essential vitamins and minerals.

Smoothies and Juices:

Make hydrating smoothies or juices using water-rich fruits and vegetables. Add ingredients like watermelon, cucumber, and citrus fruits to create refreshing and hydrating beverages. You can also incorporate plant-based protein sources, like pea protein, to enhance nutritional value.

Monitor Sweat Loss:

Be aware of your sweat loss during exercise, especially in hot and humid conditions. Weigh yourself before and after workouts to estimate fluid loss. Aim to drink about 16-20 ounces of water for every pound lost during exercise.

Pre-Exercise Hydration:

Ensure you are well-hydrated before starting any physical activity. Drink water throughout the day and consider consuming hydrating foods, like fruits, before exercise. Avoid excessive caffeine intake, as it can have diuretic effects.

Post-Exercise Rehydration:

After workouts, rehydrate with water or a hydrating beverage. Consider including electrolyte-rich foods or beverages if the exercise session has been intense or prolonged. A post-workout smoothie with water-rich fruits and vegetables can be a hydrating and nutritious choice.

Hydration with Meals:

Drink water with your meals to stay adequately hydrated. Sometimes, increased fiber intake from a plant-based diet may require additional water to aid digestion.

Listen to Your Body:

Pay attention to your body's signals for thirst. Thirst is a natural indicator that your body needs water. Additionally, monitor the color of your urine;

pale yellow is generally a sign of adequate hydration.

Consider Personalized Hydration Plans:

Consult with a sports nutritionist or dietitian to create a personalized hydration plan based on your individual needs, considering factors such as training intensity, duration, and environmental conditions.

Chapter 6

Plant-powered celebratory meals

Plant-powered celebratory meals celebrate the richness and diversity of plant-based ingredients, offering a delicious and satisfying experience for vegans. Whether you're hosting a special occasion or attending a festive gathering, plant-powered celebratory meals can be vibrant, flavorful, and nutritionally satisfying.

 Here's an overview:

Appetizers:

Stuffed Mushrooms:

Mushrooms filled with a mixture of breadcrumbs, herbs, and vegan cheese.

Vegan Spring Rolls:

Rice paper wraps filled with fresh veggies, tofu, and a dipping sauce.

Guacamole and Salsa:

A classic combo of mashed avocados with tomatoes, onions, cilantro, and lime, paired with a fresh tomato salsa.

Main Courses:

Roasted Vegetable Tart:

A flaky pastry filled with a medley of roasted vegetables and a savory plant-based cream.

Vegan Lasagna:

Layers of pasta, rich tomato sauce, vegan cheese, and a variety of sautéed vegetables.

Stuffed Bell Peppers:

Bell peppers filled with a mix of quinoa, black beans, corn, and spices.

Mushroom Risotto:

Creamy risotto made with Arborio rice, mushrooms, and vegetable broth.
Sides:

Maple Glazed Brussels Sprouts:

Brussels sprouts roasted with maple syrup, balsamic vinegar, and a sprinkle of nuts.

Garlic Mashed Potatoes:

Creamy mashed potatoes made with garlic, plant-based milk, and vegan butter.

Quinoa Salad with Pomegranate:

A refreshing salad with quinoa, arugula, pomegranate seeds, and a citrus vinaigrette.

Desserts:

Vegan Chocolate Cake:

Moist chocolate cake layered with vegan chocolate ganache.

Coconut Mango Sorbet:

A refreshing and dairy-free sorbet made with coconut milk and ripe mangoes.

Berry Parfait:

Layers of mixed berries, coconut yogurt, and granola.

Beverages:

Sparkling Fruit Punch:

A bubbly mix of fruit juices, soda, and fresh fruit slices.

Herb-Infused Lemonade:

Lemonade infused with basil, mint, or rosemary for a unique twist.

Here are some other desserts that can be made for such wonderful events.

Vegan Chocolate Avocado Mousse:

Ingredients:
Ripe avocados
Cocoa powder
Maple syrup or agave
Vanilla extract

Instructions:

Blend ripe avocados, cocoa powder, maple syrup or agave, and vanilla extract until smooth.
Chill in the refrigerator before serving.

Vegan Chocolate Chip Cookies:

Ingredients:
Flour
Coconut oil
Brown sugar
Baking soda
Vegan chocolate chips

Instructions:
Mix the ingredients to form a cookie dough.
Bake until golden brown.

Vegan Berry Parfait:

Ingredients:
Mixed berries (strawberries, blueberries, raspberries)
Vegan yogurt or coconut cream
Granola

Instructions:
Layer berries, vegan yogurt or coconut cream, and granola in a glass.

<u>Vegan Peanut Butter Cups:</u>

Ingredients:

Vegan chocolate chips
Peanut butter
Coconut oil
Maple syrup

Instructions:
Melt chocolate chips with coconut oil and maple syrup.
Pour a small amount into molds, add a dollop of peanut butter, and cover with more chocolate.

<u>Vegan Coconut Bliss Balls:</u>

Ingredients:
Shredded coconut
Almond flour
Maple syrup
Vanilla extract

Instructions:
Mix ingredients, roll into balls, and refrigerate until firm.

Vegan Chocolate-Dipped Strawberries:

Ingredients:
Fresh strawberries
Vegan chocolate chips

Instructions:
Melt chocolate chips and dip strawberries.
Place on parchment paper until the chocolate
hardens.

Vegan Banana Ice Cream:

Ingredients:
Frozen bananas
Plant-based milk
Vanilla extract

Instructions:
Blend frozen bananas, plant-based milk, and vanilla
extract until creamy.
Serve immediately.

Vegan Lemon Blueberry Cheesecake Bars:

Ingredients:
Almond flour
Cashews

Lemon juice
Blueberries

Instructions:
Make a crust with almond flour, blend cashews, lemon juice, and layer with blueberries.

Vegan Apple Crisp:

Ingredients:
Apples
Oats
Maple syrup
Cinnamon

Instructions:
Slice apples, mix with oats, maple syrup, and cinnamon, and bake until golden.

Vegan Chocolate Cake:

Ingredients:
Flour
Cocoa powder
Baking soda
Sugar
Plant-based milk
Vinegar

Vanilla extract

Instructions:
Mix dry ingredients, add wet ingredients, and bake into a rich chocolate cake.
Frost with vegan chocolate ganache if desired.

Conclusion

In conclusion, embarking on a high-protein diet journey can be both exciting and beneficial, offering a path to improved health, fitness, and overall well-being. The recipes and insights shared in this high-protein diet cookbook for beginners provide a foundation for individuals eager to explore the world of nutritious and protein-packed meals. From hearty breakfast options to satisfying main courses and delectable snacks, this cookbook encourages a wholesome approach to achieving protein goals while enjoying a diverse range of flavors.

Balanced diet

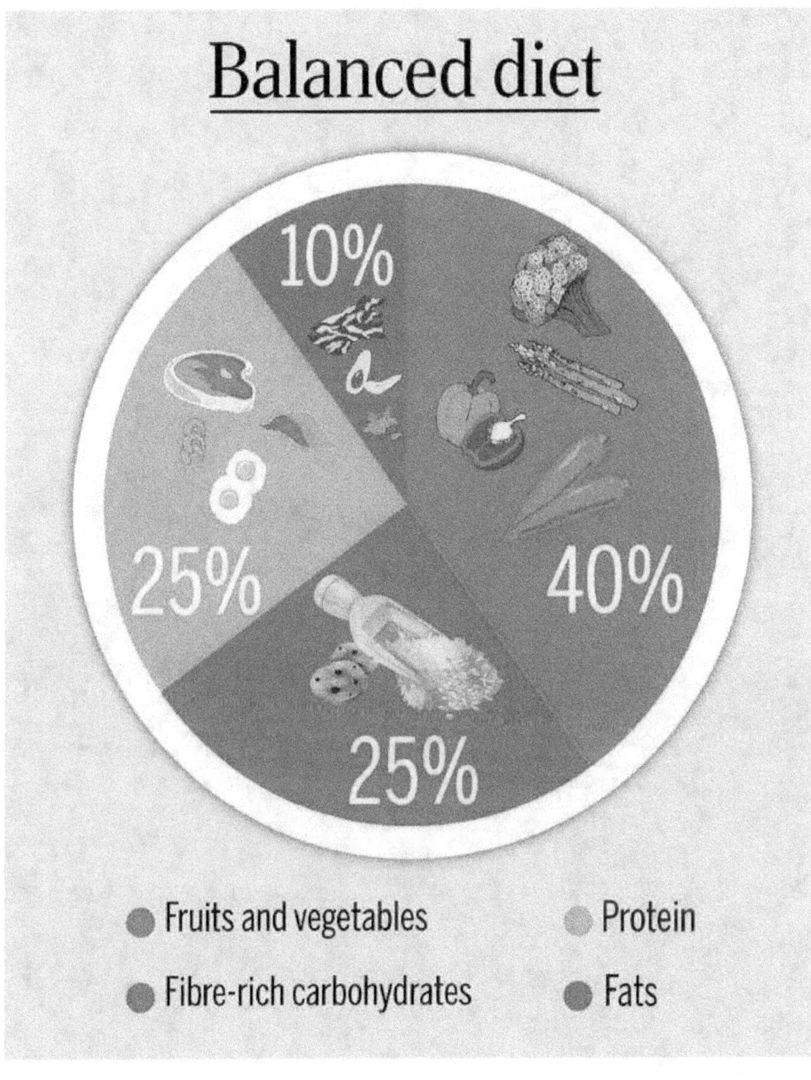